SIMPLY ALKALINE COOKBOOK FOR BEGINNERS

31 Easy Recipes to Improve your Internal and External Health by Cleansing Liver and Kidneys and Restoring Balance in your Body

BY

Phoebe Hall

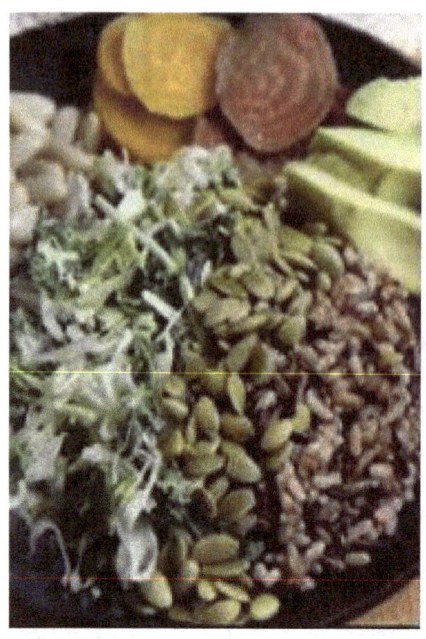
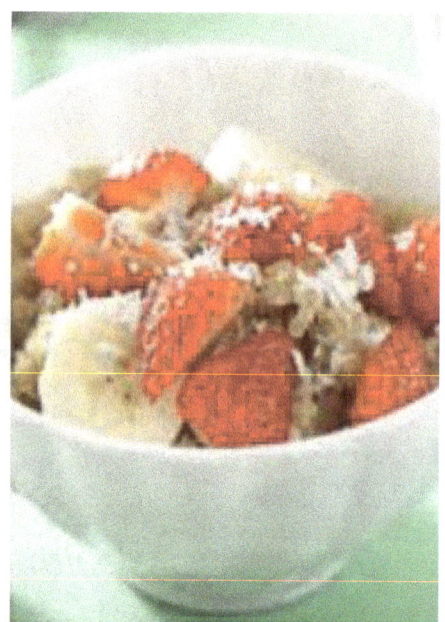
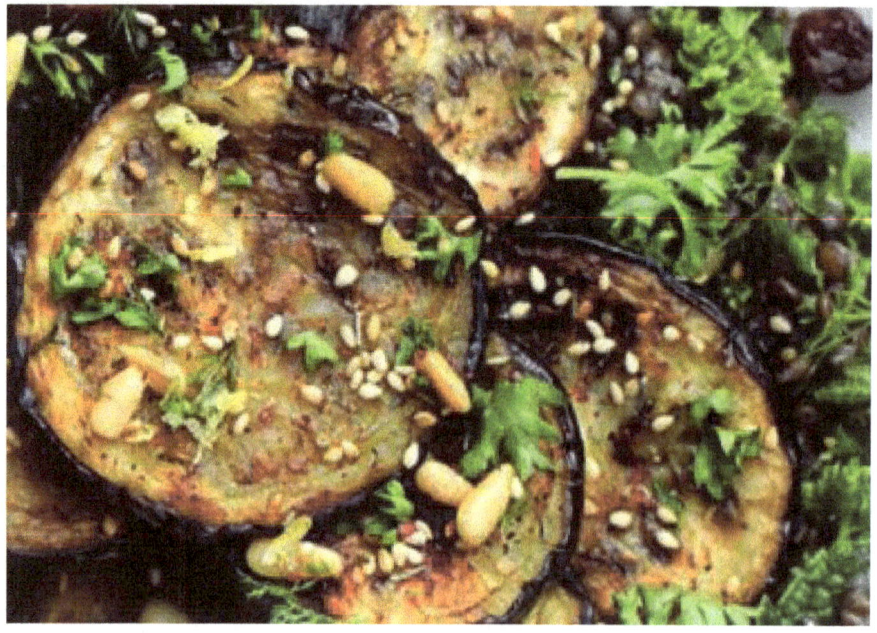

© Copyright 2021 - All rights reserved.

The content contained within this book may not be reproduced, duplicated or transmitted without direct written permission from the author or the publisher.

Under no circumstances will any blame or legal responsibility be held against the publisher, or author, for any damages, reparation, or monetary loss due to the information contained within this book. Either directly or indirectly.

Legal Notice:

This book is copyright protected. This book is only for personal use. You cannot amend, distribute, sell, use, quote or paraphrase any part, or the content within this book, without the consent of the author or publisher.

Disclaimer Notice:

Please note the information contained within this document is for educational and entertainment purposes only. All effort has been executed to present accurate, up to date, and reliable, complete information. No warranties of any kind are declared or implied. Readers acknowledge that the author is not engaging in the rendering of legal, financial, medical or professional advice. The content within this book has been derived from various sources.

Please consult a licensed professional before attempting any techniques outlined in this book. By reading this document, the reader agrees that under no circumstances is the author responsible for any losses, direct or indirect, which are incurred as a result of the use of information contained within this document, including, but not limited to, errors, omissions, or inaccuracies.

Table of Contents

Introduction --------------------------------------8

1. Almond & Polenta Skillet ---------------------10
2. Vegetable Tagine With Almonds --------------12
3. Almond Crumble Slice -------------------------14
4. Berry Almond Bakewell ------------------------17
5. Lemon & Mint Aubergine Tagine With Almond Couscous --20
6. Barley Risotto -----------------------------------23
7. Baked Cauliflower With Almond Crumbs -----25
8. Coconut & Jam Macaroon Traybake ----------28
9. Coconut Dhal & Chickpeas--------------------30
10. Snowy Coconut--------------------------------33
11. Coconut Macaroons --------------------------36
12. Coconut & Banana Pancakes ----------------38
13. Coconut French Toast With Spiced Roasted Pineapple--40
14. Coconut Steamed Sponge --------------------43
15. Choc & Coconut Traybake -------------------46
16. Coconut & Squash ----------------------------49
17. Coconut Creams With Mango & Lime --------52
18. Coconut Chai Traybake ----------------------55
19. Sweet Potato, Coconut & Lemongrass Soup With Coriander Sambal ---------------------------58
20. Coconut Custard Tart With Roasted Pineapple---61
21. Coconut & Banana Smoothie -----------------65

22. Sri Lankan Braised Roots Stew & Coconut Dhal Dumplings -- 68
23. Matcha & Coconut Trees ---------------------- 72
24. Black Dhal -------------------------------------- 75
25. Tarka Dhal -------------------------------------- 78
26. Potato Dhal With Curried Vegetables --------- 80
27. Black Dhal With Crispy Onions ---------------- 84
28. Mild Split Pea & Spinach Dhal ---------------- 87
29. Makhani Dhal ---------------------------------- 90
30. Tomatoes Stuffed With Fruity Dhal ----------- 92
31. Halloumi Fritters With Coriander Dip --------- 94

Conclusion -- **97**

INTRODUCTION

With regards to improving bone wellbeing, next to no you do matters more than improving your corrosive alkaline offset with an alkaline eating plan. Regardless of whether you exercise and breaking point poisons, if your corrosive alkaline equilibrium is wrong, you'll in any case have superfluous bone misfortune over the long haul. An alkaline diet is a fundamental piece of normal bone wellbeing.

Here are some broad rules for eating alkaline:

Zero in on eating entire food varieties, similar to vegetables, root crops, natural products, nuts, seeds, flavors, entire grains and beans (particularly lentils).

Drink alkalizing refreshments like spring water and ginger root or green tea, water with the juice of an entire lemon or lime.

Eat more modest measures of fundamental fats, meat, fish, pasta and different grains.

Dispose of handled and fake food sources, caffeine, white sugar, and white flour.

Try not to be hesitant to utilize genuine spread, ghee, and full-fat milk (in the event that you use dairy).

Dress servings of mixed greens or cook with top notch fats like cold-squeezed virgin olive oil, coconut oil, and avocado oil.

1. Almond & polenta skillet

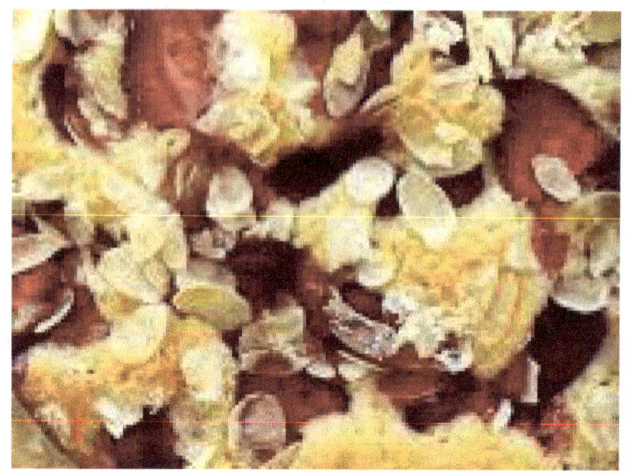

Prep:15 mins Cook:40 mins Easy Serves 4 – 6

Ingredients:

- 170g unsalted spread, softened, in addition to extra for the skillet
- 170g golden caster sugar
- 1 tsp vanilla bean paste or concentrate
- ½ tsp almond remove
- 2 eggs, at room temperature
- 120g self-raising flour
- 60g fine polenta
- 60g ground almonds
- 150g strawberries, diced
- vanilla frozen yogurt or coagulated cream, to serve

Strategy:

1. Spread a 20cm griddle or cake tin with a little margarine. Heat the oven to 180C/160C fan/gas 4.
2. Beat together the softened margarine, sugar, vanilla and almond separate for 5 mins, or until light and feathery. Add the eggs, each in turn, blending after every option to join, at that point crease through the flour, polenta and ground almonds. Overlay through a large portion of the strawberries.
3. Spoon the combination into the skillet or cake tin and smooth over. Dab with the excess strawberries and heat for 40-45 mins or until golden brown and firm. Serve warm with frozen yogurt or thickened cream.

2. Vegetable tagine with almonds

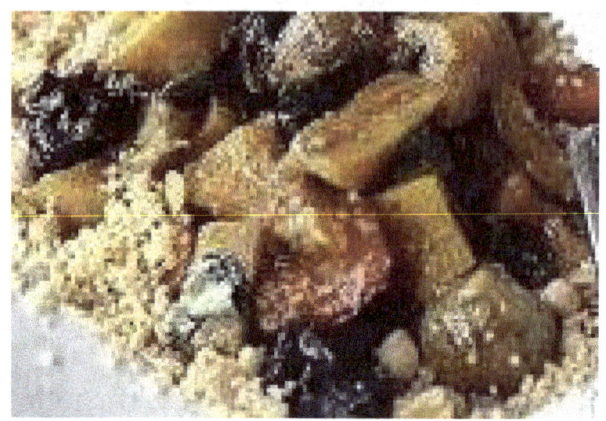

Prep:20 mins Cook:15 mins Ready in 35 mins Easy Serves 4

Ingredients:

- 400g pack shallot , stripped and cut down the middle
- 2 tbsp olive oil
- 1 large butternut squash , about 1.25kg/2 lb 12oz, stripped, deseeded and cut into scaled down lumps
- 1 tsp ground cinnamon
- ½ tsp ground ginger
- 450ml solid seasoned vegetable stock
- 12 little hollowed prunes
- 2 tsp clear nectar
- 2 red peppers , deseeded and cut into pieces

- 3 tbsp chopped coriander
- 2 tbsp chopped mint , in addition to extra for spinkling
- For the couscous
- 250g couscous
- 1 tbsp harissa (Moroccan stew paste)
- 400g can chickpea , washed and depleted
- small bunch toasted chipped almonds

Strategy:

1. Fry the shallots in the oil for 5 mins until they are mellowing and browned. Add the squash and flavors, and mix for 1 min. Pour in the stock, season well, at that point add the prunes and nectar. Cover and stew for 8 mins.
2. Add the peppers and cook for 8-10 mins until simply delicate. Mix in the coriander and mint.
3. Pour 400ml bubbling water over the couscous in a bowl, at that point mix in the harissa with ½ tsp salt. Tip in the chickpeas, at that point cover and leave for 5 mins. Cushion up with a fork and present with the tagine, chipped almonds and additional mint.

3. Almond crumble slice

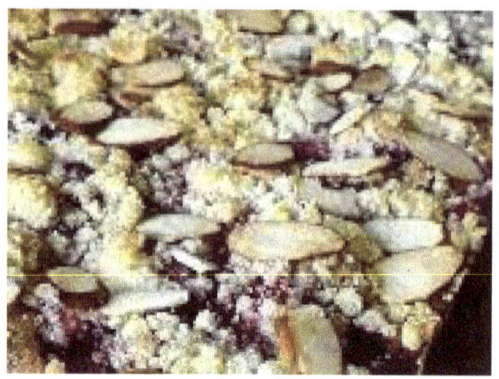

Prep:15 mins Cook:1 hr and 5 mins Plus cooling
More effort Cuts into 16 slices

Ingredients:
- 250g pack spread (this should be freezing)
- 225g caster sugar
- 300g ground almond
- 140g plain flour , in addition to 25g/1oz
- 2 eggs
- 1 tsp cinnamon
- 1 tsp preparing powder
- approx 6 plums , stoned and cut into sixths
- 50g chipped almond

Strategy:
1. Heat oven to 180C/fan 160C/gas 4. Spread and line a 20 x 30cm preparing tin with heating paper. Put the spread, sugar and

ground almonds into a food processor, at that point beat until the combination looks like unpleasant breadcrumbs. Spoon out a large portion of the blend into a bowl and put away.

2. Add 140g flour in with the general mish-mash in the processor and whizz until it simply frames a mixture. Tip into the tin and press down with the rear of a spoon. Prepare for 15-20 mins until golden. Leave to cool for 10 mins.
3. To make the filling, put the excess spread and the sugar and almond blend once more into the processor, saving a couple tbsp for the fixing. Add the eggs, the 25g flour, cinnamon and preparing powder and whizz to a delicate hitter. Spread over the base.
4. Top with the plum pieces and some additional caster sugar and cinnamon. Prepare for 20 mins, at that point sprinkle with the leftover disintegrate blend and chipped almonds. Cook for another 20 mins or until golden. Leave to cool in the tin prior to cutting.
5. **Formula TIPS**
6. MAKE IT BY HAND

7. On the off chance that you don't have a food processor, rub the ingredients for Step 1 along with your fingers. Pop the bowl in the ice chest for 10 mins if the spread turns oily. For the remainder of the formula, utilize a couple of electric blenders, or a wooden spoon and a blending bowl.

4. Berry almond Bakewell

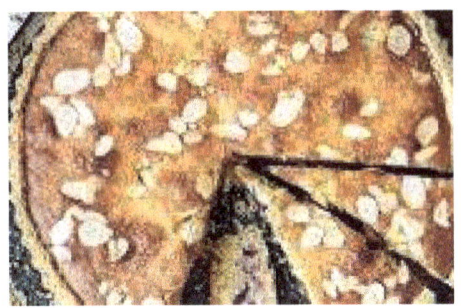

Prep:30 mins Cook:45 mins plus chilling Easy cuts into 12 slices

Ingredients:
- 400g shortcrust baked good cut from a 500g square
- 100g just-defrosted frozen raspberries
- 25g chipped almonds
- For the frangipane wipe
- 75g self-raising flour , in addition to some extra for cleaning
- 75g ground almonds
- 150g Total Sweet (xylitol)
- 150g softened spread
- 1 tsp preparing powder
- ½ tsp almond extricate
- 3 large eggs

Strategy:

1. Daintily carry out the baked good on a softly floured surface , at that point use it to line the base and sides of a 25cm non-stick, free based tart tin. You can leave a little shade of baked good, however cut back any perceptible overabundance. Prick the base with a fork and chill for 20 mins. Heat oven to 200C/180C fan/gas 6 and put a preparing sheet inside to heat up.
2. Line the baked good case with preparing material, load up with preparing beans and cook on the hot sheet for 10 mins – the eruption of heat from the heating sheet will assist with forestalling a soaked base. Cautiously lift off the paper with the beans and heat for 3 mins more to cook the cake base. Turn down the oven to 180C/160C fan/gas 4.
3. For the frangipane, put every one of the ingredients in a large bowl and beat with an electric rush until well blended (on the other hand, barrage in a food processor). Disperse the raspberries into the baked good case, spoon over the almond blend and smooth the top with a blade. Disperse over the chipped

almonds and heat for 30-40 mins until golden and firm. Cautiously trim any overabundance baked good from the edge of the tart with a sharp blade prior to serving.
4. GOES WELL WITH
5. Exemplary vanilla frozen yogurt
6. Espresso mixed drinks
7. Salted almond weak

5. Lemon & mint aubergine tagine with almond couscous

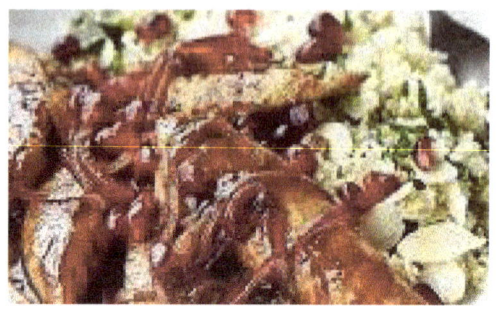

Preparation and cooking time Prep:25 mins Cook:25 mins Easy Serves 4

Ingredients:

- 1 tbsp rapeseed oil
- 1 large onion , chopped
- 3 garlic cloves , chopped
- 1 tbsp harissa
- 1 tsp cumin seeds
- ½ tsp ground cinnamon
- 200ml diminished salt vegetable stock
- 400g can chopped tomato
- 350g child aubergine , managed and a few times
- 2 strips lemon zing , finely chopped
- 390g can margarine bean , depleted

- 175g wholemeal couscous
- 40g toasted chipped almond
- 150g pot 0% fat probiotic regular yogurt, blended in with ½ squashed garlic clove and 2 tbsp chopped mint, in addition to leaves to embellish (optional)

Technique:
1. Heat the oil in a large non-stick dish and fry the onion and garlic for 5 mins. Mix in the harissa, cumin and cinnamon, cook momentarily, at that point tip in the stock and tomatoes.
2. Add the aubergines and lemon, at that point cover the container and cook delicately for 15-20 mins until the aubergines are meltingly delicate. Add the spread beans and warm through.
3. In the mean time, cook the couscous adhering to pack guidelines, at that point mix in the almonds. Serve the aubergine tagine on the couscous with the yogurt sprinkled over, and embellish with mint leaves, on the off chance that you like.
4. GOES WELL WITH

5. Moroccan cooked vegetable soup
6. Butternut and harissa hummus

6. Barley risotto

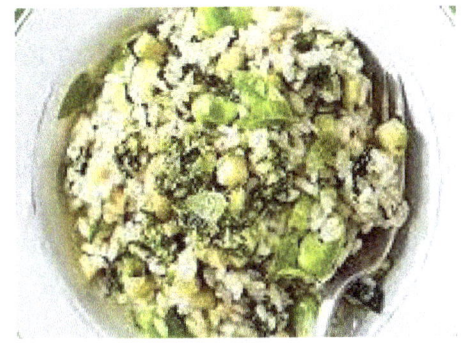

Prep:25 mins Cook:45 mins Easy Serves 2

Ingredients:

- 2 tbsp olive oil
- 1 little onion , finely chopped
- 2 large garlic cloves , squashed
- 150g pearl grain
- 700-800ml hot vegetable stock
- 250g frozen wide beans , podded, thawed out
- 1 lemon , zested
- 1 tbsp finely chopped mint , in addition to extra to serve
- 3 tbsp ricotta
- 1 tbsp finely chopped basil
- 2 tbsp parmesan or veggie lover elective, ground, in addition to extra to serve

Technique:
1. Heat the oil in a large pan. Add the onion alongside a spot of salt and tenderly fry for 8-10 mins or until softened. Mix through the garlic and cook for 1 min. Tip in the pearl grain and 600ml of the stock. Bring to the bubble, lower to a stew and cook for 35 mins, mixing routinely, until essentially all the fluid has been ingested and the pearl grain is delicate. Add the excess stock, a sprinkle at an at once, in the event that it looks excessively thick.
2. Generally hack half of the podded expansive beans (or heartbeat a couple of times in a food processor), keeping the rest entirety. Mix every one of the expansive beans into the risotto alongside the lemon zing, mint, ricotta, basil and parmesan (with a sprinkle more stock or water in the event that it looks dry). Season, at that point serve in bowls with additional mint and parmesan dispersed over.

7. Baked cauliflower with almond crumbs

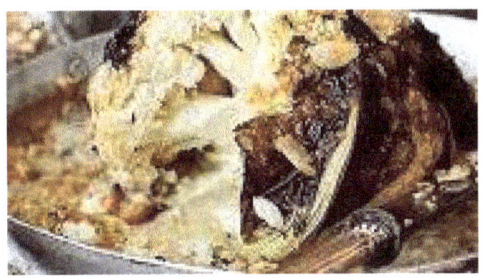

Prep:15 mins Cook:2 hrs Easy Serves 4

Ingredients:

- 1 large cauliflower, external leaves managed
- 4 tbsp rapeseed oil
- 2 onions, finely chopped
- 3 garlic cloves, squashed
- ½ tsp ground mace
- 4 thyme twigs, leaves picked from 2, 2 remaining entirety
- 4 tbsp plain flour
- 750ml unsweetened almond milk
- 150ml soya cream
- 1 tbsp wholegrain mustard
- 25g dried breadcrumbs (guarantee vegetarian well disposed, if necessary)
- 2 tbsp chipped almonds

- vegetarian garlic bread and a green serving of mixed greens with a lemony dressing, to serve

Technique:
1. Heat the oven to 180C/160C fan/gas 4. Remove enough of the cauliflower tail so it sits level, at that point cut a profound cross in the foundation of the tail. Sit the cauliflower on a piece of foil, at that point rub more than 1 tbsp oil. Sprinkle more than 2 tbsp water, season well, at that point cover firmly with the foil, fixing the water and cauliflower inside the bundle. Put in a heating dish and cook for 1 hr 30 mins.
2. Then, cook the onions with a touch of salt and 2 tbsp oil in a container until delicate and clear. Mix in the garlic, mace, thyme leaves and flour and mix for 2 mins, at that point add the almond milk. Bring to a stew, mixing, at that point season. When somewhat thickened, eliminate from the heat and mix in the soya cream and mustard.
3. Rub the breadcrumbs with the leftover oil. Mix in the almonds.

4. Uncover the cauliflower and get back to the dish. Pour the sauce everywhere on the cauliflower and into the dish. Dissipate the scraps on top, and tear over the two entire thyme branches. Turn the oven up to 200C/180C fan/gas 6. Prepare for 15-20 mins more, until the sauce is percolating and thickened marginally, and the pieces and cauliflower are golden. Cut into wedges and present with a green serving of mixed greens and some garlic bread.
5. GOES WELL WITH
6. Potato, shredded fledgling and chestnut gratin
7. Winter greens, pecan and sage lasagne
8. Spiced beet and red spelt pie with horseradish baked goo

8. Coconut & jam macaroon traybake

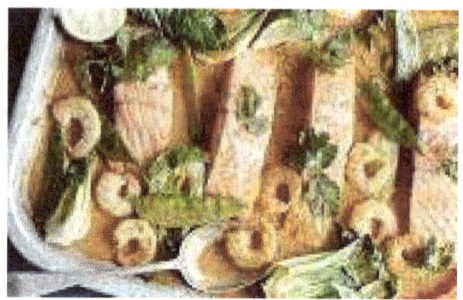

Preparation and cooking time Prep:15 mins Cook:30 mins plus chilling Easy Makes 16-20

Ingredients:

- 250g caster sugar
- 4 egg whites , beaten
- 1 tsp vanilla concentrate
- 300g dried up coconut
- 25g plain flour
- 200g raspberry jam
- 100g dull chocolate , chopped

Strategy:

1. Line a 20 x 30cm preparing tin with heating material. Heat the oven to 180C/160C fan/gas 4.
2. Blend the sugar, egg whites, vanilla and a touch of salt together in a bowl. Add the

coconut and flour and mix until completely joined – the blend will be very thick and tacky. Tip into the tin and tenderly spread out with a spatula. Spot the jam over the top using a teaspoon, nestling it into the player. Heat for 25-30 mins, until set and golden around the edges. Leave to cool totally in the tin.
3. Soften the chocolate in the microwave, or in a bowl set over a container of stewing water. Eliminate the cake from the tin, shower with chocolate and leave to set prior to cutting into squares. Will keep in an impermeable holder for as long as seven days.
4. GOES WELL WITH
5. Cultivated cheddar and chive pancakes
6. Smooth bacon and tomato pasta salad
7. Curried rice and egg salad

9. coconut dhal & chickpeas

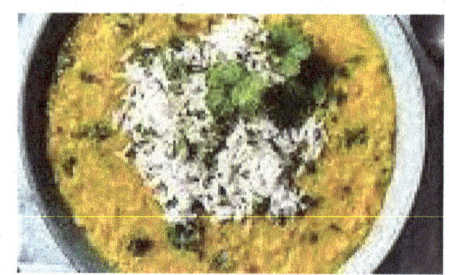

Prep:15 mins Cook:50 mins Easy Serves 4-6

Ingredients:

- 1½ tbsp ghee or groundnut oil
- 2 onions , finely chopped
- 8 garlic cloves , finely chopped
- 3cm piece ginger , stripped and ground
- 1 tsp ground turmeric
- 1 tbsp nigella seeds
- 2 tsp ground cumin
- 1 tsp ground coriander
- 1 tsp paprika
- 1 cinnamon stick
- ½ tsp stew pieces
- 4 cardamom units , seeds eliminated and ground
- 2 sound leaves
- 2 x 400g jars chickpeas , depleted

- 75g yellow split peas
- 400ml would coconut be able to drain
- For the trimming
- 2 tbsp ghee , or unsalted spread
- 2 shallots , finely cut
- 1 tbsp cumin seeds
- 1 tsp dark mustard seeds
- ½ tsp stew chips
- 3 tbsp coriander leaves , chopped

Strategy:

1. Heat the ghee or groundnut oil and fry the onion over a medium heat until it's pale gold and delicate. Add the garlic and ginger and cook for two or three mins. Mix in every one of the flavors and cook for one more moment or thereabouts, at that point add every one of the excess ingredients and 450ml water. Bring to simply underneath edge of boiling over, turn the heat down and stew for around 40 mins until the split peas are delicate. On the off chance that you like your dhal thick in surface, pound the chickpeas to separate them. In the event that the combination is getting dry, add more water. On the off chance that it's

excessively slender, continue to cook until you get the thickness you need. There is no 'correct' consistency; dhal can be nearly brothy or like a thick purée.

2. To serve, heat the ghee or spread in a container and add the shallots. Fry until they're golden, at that point add the cumin seeds, dark mustard seeds and stew pieces. Cook until their smells are delivered. Dissipate coriander on top of the dhal, at that point pour over the spiced spread.

10. Snowy coconut

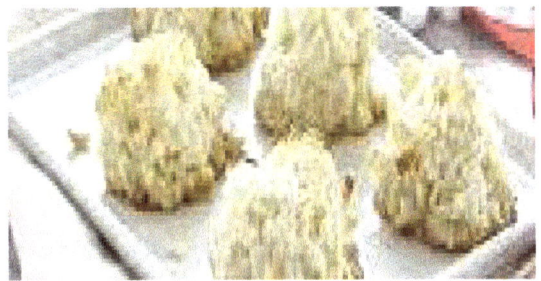

Prep:20 mins Cook:1 hr and 10 mins Easy Serves 10

Ingredients:

- 185g margarine softened, in addition to extra for the tin
- 185g coconut milk, whisked
- 250g caster sugar
- 250g self-raising flour
- 3 large eggs
- 1 tsp coconut extricate (optional)
- 25g dried up coconut
- For the icing
- 100g spread, softened
- 250g icing sugar
- 2 tbsp coconut milk
- ½ tsp coconut extricate (optional)
- 25g coconut chips or dried up coconut

- white chocolate truffles or large white sprinkles, to enliven (optional)

Strategy:

1. Heat the oven to 180C/160C fan/gas 4. Spread a 900g portion tin (our own deliberate 10 x 21 x 5cm) and line the base with a long piece of preparing material that overhangs the sides.

2. Put the spread, coconut milk, sugar, flour, eggs, coconut extricate (if using) and dried up coconut in a large bowl and beat with an electric speed until consolidated. Scratch into the readied tin and level the top with a spatula or the rear of a spoon. Heat for 55 mins-1 hr, or until the cake is risen and golden brown and a stick embedded into the center confesses all. In the event that any wet cake combination sticks to the stick, prepare for another 5-10 mins, at that point check once more. Leave to cool in the tin for 10 mins, at that point lift the cake out onto a wire rack, using the material to help you. Leave to cool totally. The cooled cake will keep in the cooler, well wrapped, for as long as two months.

3. To make the icing, beat the spread, sugar, coconut milk and coconut separate, if using, in a bowl until smooth and velvety. Spread over the highest point of the cake using a range blade or the rear of a spoon, at that point dissipate over a liberal layer of coconut chips. Enhance with white chocolate truffle 'snowballs' or large white sprinkles, in the event that you like.
4. **Tips:**
5. Use sprouted bread which is high in alkalinity

11. Coconut macaroons

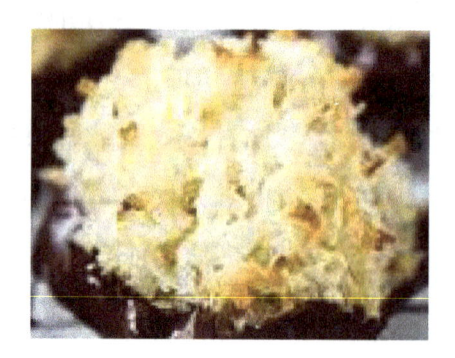

Prep:30 mins Cook:15 mins plus cooling Easy Makes 10-12

Ingredients:

- 80g caster sugar
- 150g dried up coconut
- 1 tsp vanilla paste
- 90g dull chocolate

Strategy:

1. Whisk together the egg whites and caster sugar in a large bowl for 2-3 mins until light and foamy, and the sugar has disintegrated. Add the coconut, a spot of salt and the vanilla, at that point mix until joined. Leave to represent 10 mins.
2. Heat the oven to 170C/150C fan/gas 3½. Line a preparing sheet with heating material. Scoop teaspoonfuls of the combination and fold into

minimal balls, at that point organize on the readied heating sheet. Prepare for 10-12 mins until golden.

3. Leave on the heating sheet to cool totally. Dissolve the chocolate in a heatproof bowl over a dish of stewing water, ensuring the bowl doesn't contact the water, or in short 20-second barges in the microwave. Tip the dissolved chocolate into a little bowl, at that point plunge the lower part of each cooled macaroon into the chocolate and wipe off any overabundance. Organize on a sheet of preparing material, chocolate-side up, at that point put in the refrigerator for 20 mins, or until set. You can utilize any leftover liquefied chocolate to pipe in crisscrosses over the top, in the event that you like, leave to set.

12. Coconut & banana pancakes

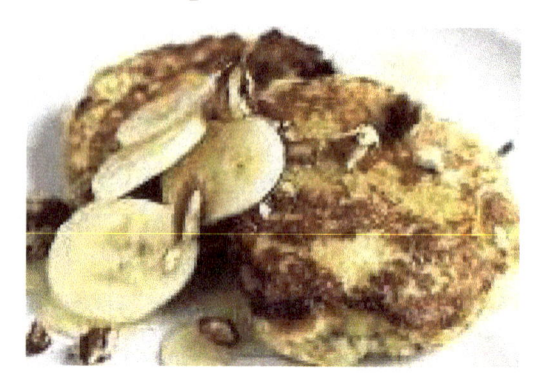

Prep:10 mins Cook:15 mins Easy Serves 8 – 10

Ingredients:
- 150g plain flour
- 2 tsp heating powder
- 3 tbsp golden caster sugar
- 400ml would coconut be able to drain, shaken well
- vegetable oil, for fricasseeing
- 1-2 bananas, meagerly cut
- 2 enthusiasm organic products, substance scooped out

Strategy:
1. Filter the flour and preparing powder into a bowl, and mix in 2 tbsp of the sugar and a touch of salt. Empty the coconut milk into a

bowl, rush to blend in any fat that has isolated, at that point measure out 300ml into a container. Mix the milk gradually into the flour combination to make a smooth hitter, or whizz everything in a blender.

2. Heat a shallow skillet or level frying pan and brush it with oil. Utilize 2 tbsp of hitter to make every flapjack, browning two all at once – any more will make it hard to flip them. Drive 4-5 bits of banana into every flapjack and cook until bubbles begin to fly on a superficial level, and the edges look dry. They will be somewhat more fragile than egg-based flapjacks, so turn them over cautiously and cook different sides for 1 min. Rehash to make 8-10 flapjacks.

3. In the mean time, put the excess coconut milk and sugar in a little skillet. Add a spot of salt and stew until the blend thickens to the consistency of single cream. Utilize this as a sauce for the flapjacks and spoon over a portion of the energy organic product seeds.

13. Coconut French toast with spiced roasted pineapple

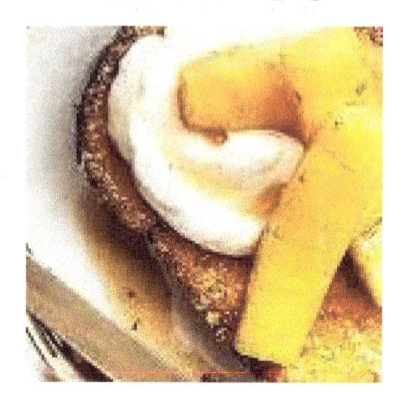

Prep:25 mins Cook:25 mins Serves 2

Ingredients:

- 150ml coconut milk
- ½ tsp vanilla concentrate
- 2 thick cuts brioche
- handle of spread (about 20g)
- 2 tbsp parched coconut
- plain or coconut yogurt, to serve
- For the pineapple
- ½ little pineapple
- 1½ tbsp maple syrup
- touch of ground allspice

Strategy:

1. Whisk the eggs, coconut milk and vanilla together in a wide, shallow bowl. Dunk the brioche cuts into the combination, allowing each to sit in the bowl for 1-2 mins on each side to absorb the fluid. The blend ought to be totally consumed by the brioche prior to cooking.
2. Heat the oven to 200C/180C fan/gas 6. To set up the pineapple, remove the skin, leaves and any eyes, at that point cut the tissue into long, stout pieces (you'll need around three for each individual). Remove the extreme center and dispose of. Spot the pineapple pieces in a little heating dish, shower over the maple syrup and sprinkle with allspice. Cook for 15 mins, turning part of the way through and brushing with the tacky syrup in the dish.
3. In the interim, dissolve the margarine in a griddle over a low-medium heat until frothing. Dissipate the parched coconut over a plate, and plunge in each side of the splashed brioche cuts to cover. (The bread will be fragile, so do this cautiously.) Cook the brioche cuts for 3-4 mins on each side until golden and cooked through. Split between two plates, at that

point top each with a touch of yogurt, three of the cooked pineapple pieces, at that point shower over any juices from the simmering tin.

4. GOES WELL WITH
5. Smoked salmon pâté with tear and offer brioche buns
6. Curried margarine prepared cod with cauliflower and chickpeas
7. One-skillet herby broil sheep with lemon, potatoes & feta

14. coconut steamed sponge

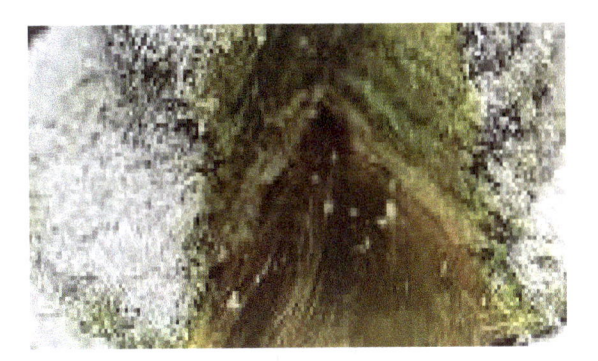

Prep:15 mins Cook:1 hr plus freezing Easy Serves 6

Ingredients:

- 175g unsalted spread , softened, in addition to extra for the bowls
- 6 tbsp raspberry jam
- 175g caster sugar
- 3 large eggs
- 150g self-raising flour
- 25g dried up coconut , blitzed in a little food processor until fine
- 1 tsp vanilla concentrate
- 2 tbsp coconut cream , in addition to 2 tbsp to serve (optional)
- 500g thick custard , to serve

Technique:

1. Spread six little pudding bowls and spoon 1 tbsp jam into the lower part of every one.
2. Put the margarine and sugar in a medium bowl and beat with an electric speed until pale and fleecy. Beat in one of the eggs followed by a spoonful of the flour, at that point proceed until every one of the eggs have been joined. Overlay in the leftover flour, the coconut and a touch of salt, at that point the vanilla and coconut cream. Spoon the blend into the readied bowls, leaving a 1cm hole at the top.
3. Put the bowls on a preparing plate, move to the cooler and freeze until strong. Will keep in an impenetrable holder, or firmly enveloped by the cooler for as long as a quarter of a year.
4. Heat the oven to 180C/160C fan/gas 4. Put the bowls in a profound preparing dish and half-load up with bubbled water from the pot. Firmly cover the dish with thwart and heat for 1 hr, or until a stick embedded into the center of a wipe tells the truth.
5. Warm the custard with the leftover 2 tbsp coconut cream, if using, and fill shallow dishes. Run a blade around the sides of the bowls and cautiously turn out the wipes onto the custard.

6. GOES WELL WITH
7. Fig wipe pudding
8. Extreme tacky toffee pudding
9. A definitive makeover: Sponge pudding and custard

15. choc & coconut traybake

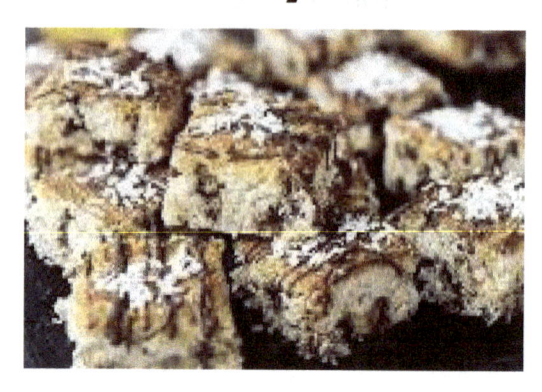

Prep:30 mins Cook:40 mins plus cooling and 1 hr 45 mins chilling Easy Makes 12 squares

Ingredients:

- 200g unsalted margarine , softened
- 100g golden caster sugar
- 100g light brown delicate sugar
- 3 large eggs
- 60g parched coconut
- 200g self-raising flour
- 100g Greek yogurt
- ½ tsp coconut enhancing (optional, see tip underneath)
- For the fixing
- 200g milk or dull chocolate , chopped into little pieces
- 200ml twofold cream

- 40g white chocolate, dissolved
- small bunch of coconut drops, toasted, or parched coconut or sprinkles

Strategy:
1. Line a 22 x 28cm rectangular cake tin with preparing material. Heat the oven to 180C/160C fan/gas 4.
2. In the first place, set up the garnish. Put the milk or dim chocolate pieces in a large heatproof bowl. Heat the twofold cream in a medium skillet until simply steaming, at that point gradually pour over the chocolate, rushing until the chocolate has liquefied and the blend is smooth. Leave to cool somewhat, at that point chill for 1 hr 30 mins until delicate, yet spoonable.
3. Beat the margarine, sugars and ¼ tsp salt together in a stand blender or using an electric speed for 5 mins, or until light and cushy. Add the eggs each in turn, beating well after every option. Add the dried up coconut, flour, yogurt and coconut seasoning, if using, and momentarily beat until just consolidated. Spoon the blend into

the tin, smooth the surface using the rear of a spoon, at that point prepare for 30 mins until golden and firm to the touch. Leave in the tin to cool totally.

4. At the point when completely cool, spread over the chocolate beating, at that point shower with the white chocolate and dissipate over the toasted coconut pieces. Chill for around 15 mins until the garnish is set. Cut into 12 squares, at that point serve.

5. **Formula TIPS**
6. WHERE TO FIND COCONUT Flavoring
7. You can discover coconut enhancing in the heating part of certain general stores, or online at expert preparing shops.

16. Coconut & squash

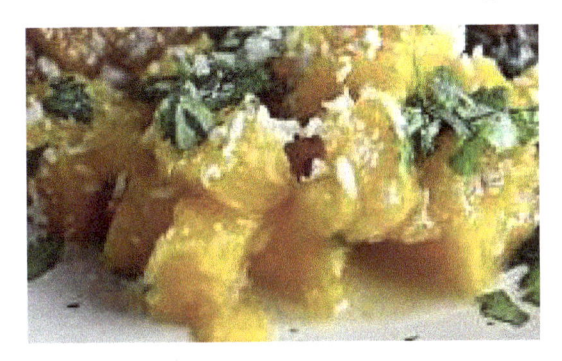

Prep:5 mins Cook:15 mins Easy Serves 4

Ingredients:
- 1 tbsp vegetable oil
- 500g butternut squash (around 1 little squash), stripped and chopped into scaled down lumps (or purchase a pack of prepared arranged to save time), see tip, underneath left
- 100g frozen chopped onions
- 4 piled tbsp gentle curry paste (we utilized korma)
- 400g can chopped tomatoes
- 400g can light coconut milk
- smaller than normal naan bread, to serve
- 400g can lentils, depleted
- 200g sack infant spinach

- 150ml coconut yogurt (we utilized Rachel's Organic), in addition to extra to serve

1. **Strategy:**

1. Heat the oil in a large dish. Put the squash in a bowl with a sprinkle of water. Cover with stick film and microwave on High for 10 mins or until delicate. In the interim, add the onions to the hot oil and cook for a couple of mins until delicate. Add the curry paste, tomatoes and coconut milk, and stew for 10 mins until thickened to a rich sauce.
2. Warm the naan breads in a low oven or in the toaster oven. Channel any fluid from the squash, at that point add to the sauce with the lentils, spinach and some flavoring. Stew for a further 2-3 mins to shrink the spinach, at that point mix in the coconut yogurt. Present with the warm naan and a spot of additional yogurt.
3. **Formula TIPS**
4. CASSIE'S TIME-SAVER
5. Cooking squash in the microwave is a lot faster than on the hob. On the off chance that you don't suffer a heart attack, cook the squash in the oven with your earlier night's dinner. You'll save time

(and cash on your energy bill), and cooked squash keeps in the refrigerator for as long as four days.

17. Coconut creams with mango & lime

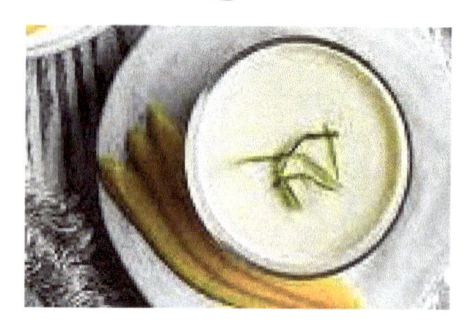

Prep:5 mins Cook:20 mins Easy Serves 4-6

Ingredient:

- 250ml coconut cream
- 300ml twofold cream
- 75g caster sugar
- ½ lime , squeezed, in addition to 4 expansive segments of zing and some fine strips, to serve (optional)
- 100g new coconut , chopped then squashed using a pestle and mortar
- 2 little gelatine leaves (about 3g) for a delicate set, or 3 leaves on the off chance that you incline toward a firmer surface
- For the mango and lime
- 1 just-ready mango
- 3 limes , squeezed

Strategy:
1. Pour the coconut cream and twofold cream into a substantial based pot with the sugar, wide portions of lime zing and squashed coconut, at that point set over a low heat, mixing a little to help the sugar disintegrate. Turn the heat off not long before it bubbles and leave to implant for 1 hr (longer is fine). Strain and discard the solids.
2. Absorb the gelatine cold water for 10 mins to mellow. Reheat the coconut combination until hand-warm (if it's too hot, the panna cotta won't set as expected). Mix in the lime juice.
3. Lift the gelatine from the water and press out the abundance fluid. Mix into the coconut combination. Split between four metal forms, each with a limit of 125ml, or up to six teacups or little dishes in case you're not turning out the panna cotta. Leave to cool, at that point put in a little cooking tin (just to move them). Cover and chill in the ice chest for around 4-6 hrs.
4. Remove the two 'cheeks' of the mango. (You could utilize the remainder of the tissue for a smoothie). Spot them, cut-side down, on a

hacking board, at that point cut on a point into slim cuts. Move to a bowl and pour the lime juice over them.

5. In the event that you need to turn out the panna cotta, plunge the molds in to a bowl of bubbling water for 5 seconds and relax the edges with a blade. For every one, put a plate over the shape, turn the form over while holding the plate set up, and shake. The panna cotta should get out. Enhancement with fine pieces of lime zing, in the event that you like. Serve close by the lime-marinated mango.

18. Coconut chai traybake

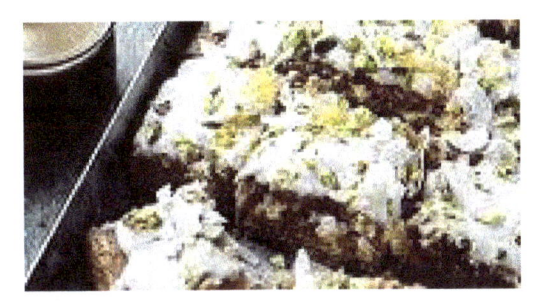

Prep:25 mins Cook:25 mins - 30 mins Easy Cuts into 15 squares

Ingredients:
- 100ml vegetable oil , in addition to a little for lubing
- 300ml coconut milk (not low-fat) - if the cream has isolated in the can, give it a decent blend prior to estimating
- 4 large eggs
- 2 tsp vanilla concentrate
- 280g light brown delicate sugar
- 250g self-raising flour
- 75g parched coconut
- 1 tsp ground ginger
- 1 tsp ground cinnamon
- ¼ nutmeg , finely ground
- ¼ tsp ground cloves

- 10 cardamom cases, seeds eliminated and squashed using a pestle and mortar
- 4 tbsp ginger syrup
- For the garnish and icing
- 3-4 tbsp coconut milk
- 140g icing sugar
- 2 balls stem ginger, finely chopped
- chopped pistachios and coconut pieces (optional)

Technique:

1. Oil a 20 x 30cm heating tin with a little oil, and line the base and favors preparing material. Heat oven to 180C/160C fan/gas 4. Measure the coconut milk and oil into a container. Break in the eggs, add the vanilla and race with a fork to consolidate.

2. In a large bowl, blend the sugar, flour, coconut, flavors and a spot of salt. Just barely get any pieces of sugar through your fingers, shaking the bowl a couple of times so they rise to the top. Pour in the wet ingredients and utilize a large speed to blend to a smooth player. Fill the tin, scratching each drop of the blend out of the bowl with a spatula.

3. Heat on the center rack of the oven for 25 mins or until a stick embedded into the center confesses all. In the event that there is any wet combination sticking to it, heat for a further 5 mins, at that point check once more. Leave to cool for 15 mins in the tin, at that point move to a wire rack and sprinkle over the ginger syrup.
4. To make the icing, blend the coconut milk with the icing sugar until smooth. Shower the icing over the cake in squiggles, at that point disperse with the chopped ginger, pistachios and coconut drops, if using. Eat warm or cold. Will save for 3 days in an impenetrable compartment.

19. Sweet potato, coconut & lemongrass soup with coriander sambal

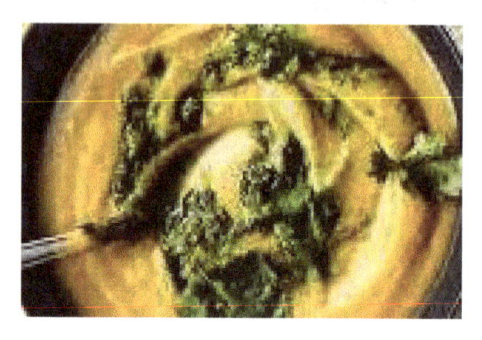

Prep:15 mins Cook:30 mins Easy Serves 4

Ingredients:

- 2 tbsp groundnut oil
- 4 spring onions , cut
- 2 large garlic cloves , cut
- 2 lemongrass stalks , external leaves eliminated and tail finely chopped
- finger-sized piece ginger , cut
- 900g yams , stripped and chopped into little pieces
- 215ml coconut milk
- 285ml vegetable stock (we utilized Bouillon)
- 1 green stew , deseeded
- 1 tsp caster sugar

- 2 limes , squeezed
- 1 little pack coriander

Technique:

1. Heat the oil in a large skillet, at that point add the spring onions, garlic, lemongrass and 3/4 of the ginger and cook for 2 mins until sweet-smelling, at that point tip in the yam. Give everything a decent blend so the yam is well covered, at that point add the coconut milk, stock and 500ml water. Bring to the bubble, at that point stew for around 25 mins until the yam is cooked through.

2. Then, tip the excess ginger, the stew, sugar, 3/4 of the lime juice and a large portion of the coriander (holding a couple of leaves for a topping) into a food processor and barrage until smooth. Move the sambal to a little container and put away.

3. Barrage the soup with a hand blender until smooth, at that point season to taste with the leftover lime juice and some salt and pepper. Split the soup among bowls and top with the coriander sambal. Topping with the held coriander leaves.

20. Coconut custard tart with roasted pineapple

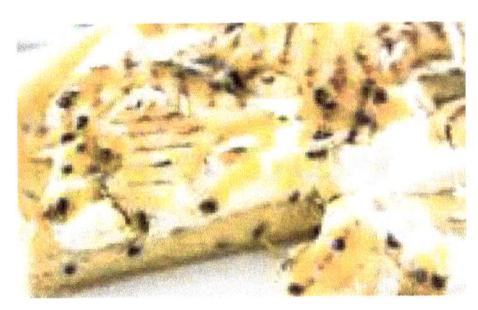

Prep:40 mins Cook:1 hr and 30 mins Plus at least 2½ hrs chilling More effort Serves 10

Ingredients:

- For the cake
- 300g plain flour , in addition to a little for cleaning
- 150g virus margarine , cut into little pieces
- 75g caster sugar
- 2 egg yolks , in addition to 1 beaten egg
- For the custard
- 400ml twofold cream
- 2 x 160ml jars coconut cream
- 3 eggs , in addition to 2 yolks
- 75g caster sugar
- new nutmeg , finely ground
- For the pineapple
- 1 little pineapple

- 4 tbsp light brown delicate sugar
- 2 tbsp rum (or use lime juice if serving to youngsters)
- new nutmeg, finely ground
- little modest bunch toasted coconut shavings, optional

Technique:

1. Rub the flour and margarine along with your fingertips until the combination looks like breadcrumbs. Add the sugar, egg yolks and 1-2 tbsp cold water, at that point blend until the mixture begins to frame clusters. Tip onto your work surface and ply a couple of times to carry any morsels into the batter. Shape into a puck, enclose by stick film and chill for at any rate 30 mins.

2. Heat oven to 180C/160C fan/gas 4 and put a preparing sheet on the center rack to heat up. Carry out the mixture on a flour-tidied surface to line the base and sides of a 23cm round fluted tart tin. Wrap it over a folding pin and lift into the tin, keeping a shade of about 1cm. Press into the corners, leaving no holes. Save the cake scraps.

3. Line the tart case with material and tip in heating beans or rice. Heat for 20-25 mins on the sheet, at that point eliminate the beans and material. Check for openings and fix them with the pieces. Set back in the oven for 5-10 mins to give it a nutty brown tone. Brush with the beaten egg and get back to the oven for 2 additional mins. While still warm, utilize a serrated blade to manage the cake to the stature of the tin. Leave to cool. Diminish oven to 140C/120C fan/gas 1.
4. Put the cream and coconut cream in a container and heat until steaming. Then, whisk the entire eggs, yolks and sugar until pale. Pour the hot cream over the eggs, rushing until the sugar has broken up. Empty through a sifter into a container.
5. Put the tart case on the preparing sheet in the oven, with the rack pulled out. Pour in the custard, using up however much you can. Sprinkle nutmeg over the top liberally and prepare for 50-55 mins until the custard is set with a little wobble when tenderly shaken. Leave to cool. Chill for in any event two hours, or as long as two days.

6. At the point when prepared to cook the pineapple, heat oven to 240C/220C fan/gas 8. Strip it using a blade to cut away the skin, at that point cut into four wedges and eliminate the center. Cut lengthways into long bits. Orchestrate over a heating plate fixed with material. Blend the sugar, rum (or lime juice) and a grinding of nutmeg, at that point paint this ridiculous. Heat for 10 mins, or until caramelized. Serve warm with the cool tart. We served our own on top with coconut shavings.

21. Coconut & banana smoothie

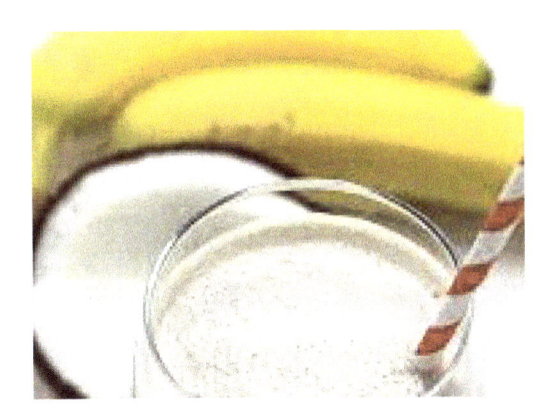

Prep:5 mins No cook Easy Serves 1

Ingredients:

- 100g coconut yogurt
- 3 tbsp milk of your decision (we utilized unsweetened almond milk)
- ½ tsp ground turmeric
- 3cm piece of new ginger, stripped
- 2 tsp baobab powder (optional)
- 1 little ready banana
- 1 tsp nectar
- 1 tbsp oats
- juice of 0.5 a lemon

Technique:

1. Add the coconut yogurt and milk to a rapid blender at that point add the turmeric, new

ginger and baobab powder (if using). Tip in the excess ingredients at that point mix until smooth. Add ice and rush again on the off chance that you lean toward a colder beverage. Fill glasses and serve.

2. **Formula TIPS**
3. Putting away YOUR SMOOTHIE
4. Is it OK to make a smoothie the other day or would it be a good idea for me to drink it straight away? Enjoying it quickly is the better choice as everything is new, however a pre-prepared smoothie is a far superior decision than a biscuit or croissant while in transit to work. In the event that you do make it the prior night you may see that the flavors change (contingent upon the ingredients), however numerous individuals favor a marginally earthier taste. A press of lemon or lime juice will help forestall oxidation and stop it going brown. Continuously cover or store it in a fixed container in the refrigerator to protect the supplements however much as could be expected. A simpler alternative, on the off chance that you realize you will be shy of time is to set up the foods grown from the ground ahead of time and freeze quickly in divide measured packs. Toward the

beginning of the day tip the frozen ingredients into the blender with your fluid and whizz.
5. MAKE IT VEGAN
6. For a vegetarian alternative, trade the nectar for a little agave nectar or maple syrup.

22. Sri Lankan braised roots stew & coconut dhal dumplings

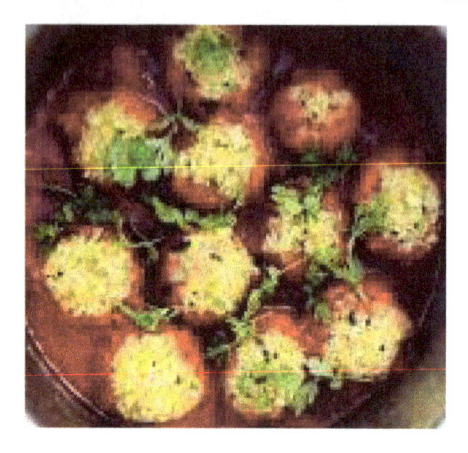

Prep:45 mins Cook:40 mins More effort Serves 4 – 6

Ingredients:
- 1 tbsp coconut oil
- 1 tsp mustard seeds
- 6 curry leaves
- 1 onion , finely cut
- 1 leek , finely cut
- 3 garlic cloves , 1 cut, 2 minced
- 2 chillies , deseeded and finely chopped
- 2 celery stem , diced
- 1 tbsp cooked curry powder (see beneath)
- 400ml can chopped tomatoes

- 2 crude beetroot , stripped and cut into implement
- 3 parsnips , cut
- 3 carrots , cut
- 400ml would coconut be able to drain
- For the dumplings
- 100g split red lentils
- 1½ tbsp coconut oil
- 1 tsp mustard seeds
- 1 tbsp curry leaves
- 75g self-raising flour
- ½ green stew , finely chopped
- ½ red onion , finely chopped
- 1 tsp turmeric
- 1 tsp red stew powder
- 80g parched coconut
- ½ lime , squeezed
- For the Sri Lankan curry powder
- 10g basmati rice
- 20g coriander seeds
- 15g cumin seeds
- 10g dark peppercorns
- 5g fenugreek seeds
- 3g cloves
- seeds from cardamom cases

- To serve
- cut spring onion
- new coriander leaves

Technique:

1. To make the curry powder: In a dry griddle, toast the rice until it's browning, at that point add every one of the flavors and toast for 3-5 mins until darkish brown yet not consumed. Rush everything in a zest processor, or pulverize with a pestle and mortar, at that point go through a strainer into a container or sealed shut holder. Will save for 2-3 weeks.
2. Heat the oil in a wok. Dissipate in the mustard seeds and curry leaves. At the point when they sizzle, add the onion, leek, garlic, bean stew, celery and a touch of salt, and cook, mixing, for 8-10 mins until the onion begins to shading. Add the curry powder and cook for 1 min more, at that point add the tomatoes, veg, coconut milk, a tsp of salt and 200ml water. Bring to the bubble, cover and stew for 10-15 mins until the veg are delicate.
3. For the dumplings, heat up the lentils in a container of water until just cooked, at that

point channel. Dissolve the coconut oil in a skillet, at that point add the mustard seeds and curry leaves and cook until sizzling. Eliminate from the heat and permit to cool marginally. Put the lentils, flour, bean stew, onion, flavors, parched coconut, lime juice and 1 tsp salt in a bowl. Blend in with your hands until joined, at that point add the coconut oil and aromatics and blend to a mixture. Structure into 12 dumplings, at that point put on top of the stew, cover with a top and cook on low for 5 mins. Top with pepper, coriander and spring onion to serve.

23. Matcha & coconut trees

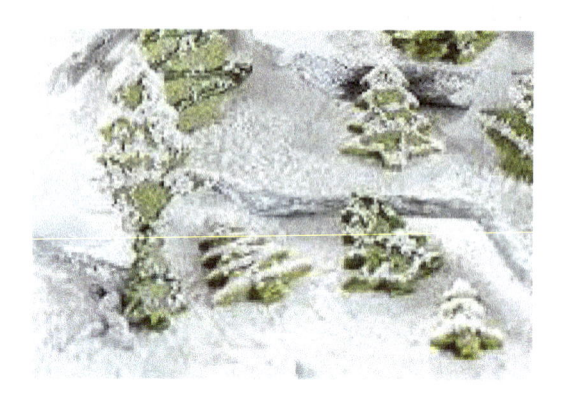

Prep:25 mins Cook:15 mins plus chilling Easy Makes about 35

Ingredients:

- 50g parched coconut , in addition to extra to embellish
- 60g icing sugar
- 150g plain flour , in addition to extra for tidying
- 2 tsp matcha powder
- 125g virus margarine , chopped
- 1 egg yolk
- 1 lime , zested and 1 tsp juice
- For the icing
- about 100g icing sugar
- around 3 tsp milk
- green food shading (optional)

- You will require
- tree-molded roll shaper

Strategy:

1. Finely crush the dried up coconut with the icing sugar in an espresso processor or food processor. Combine as one the flour and matcha powder, at that point add to the coconut combination. Add the excess ingredients and a spot of salt, and rapidly manipulate everything to a smooth mixture. Wrap and leave in the ice chest for in any event 30 mins.

2. Heat the oven to 160C/140C fan/gas 3. Carry out the batter on a floured work surface to a thickness of about 5mm and, using the tree-molded shaper, press out the trees. Put them on heating sheets fixed with preparing material and prepare for around 10-15 mins. To ensure they stay overall quite green, the trees ought to scarcely be browned. Eliminate from the oven and leave to cool.

3. For the icing, tip the icing sugar into a little bowl and continuously add the milk, mixing until smooth. Add a couple dops of food

shading, in the event that you like. Enliven the bread rolls with it, at that point sprinkle with dried up coconut. Put away until totally dry. Will keep in a hermetically sealed holder for as long as three days.

24. black dhal

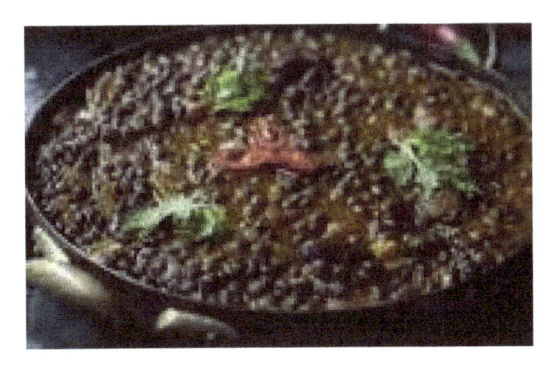

Prep:15 mins Cook:20 mins Easy Serves 4

Ingredients:

- 1 little cauliflower , cut into little florets (hold the leaves)
- 2 tsp cumin seeds
- 2 tsp turmeric
- 3 tbsp olive oil (or liquefied coconut oil)
- 1 little onion , finely chopped
- 1 tbsp garlic paste
- 1 tbsp ginger paste
- 1 red stew (deseeded on the off chance that you don't care for it excessively hot), finely chopped
- little pack coriander , stalks chopped, leaves picked to serve
- 2 x 250g pockets puy lentils
- 400ml would coconut be able to drain

- 2 limes, 1 squeezed, 1 slice into wedges to serve

Strategy:
1. Heat oven to 200C/180C fan/gas 6. Throw the cauliflower, including the leaves, with 1 tsp cumin seeds, 1 tsp turmeric and 1 tbsp oil. Season well, spread out on a preparing plate and heat for 15-20 mins or until cooked through and somewhat burned.
2. Heat 1 tbsp oil in a pot over a medium heat and add the excess flavors. When the cumin seeds start to pop, add the onion and cook for 5 mins or until softened. Mix in the garlic and ginger paste, stew, coriander stalks and 1 tbsp olive oil, and sizzle for a couple of mins until fragrant. Mix in the lentils, covering them in the flavors, at that point add the coconut milk and turn up the heat so it bubbles away. Cook for a couple of mins until the lentils have consumed a portion of the coconut milk, at that point pour in the lime squeeze and season.
3. Separation the dhal into four dishes, top with the cauliflower and a dissipating of coriander

leaves, and present with lime wedges as an afterthought.
4. GOES WELL WITH
5. Shredded chicken plate of mixed greens
6. Bombay omelet
7. Coconut fish curry traybake

25. Tarka dhal

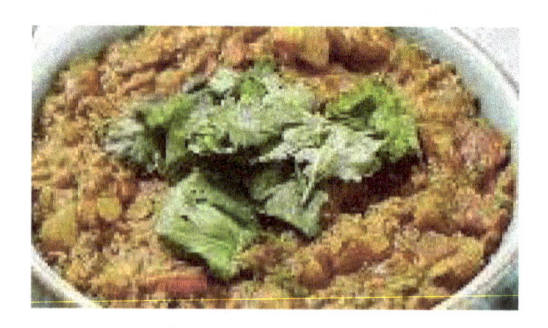

Prep:10 mins Cook:1 hr Easy Serves 2

Ingredients:

- 200g red lentils
- 2 tbsp ghee, or vegetable oil in case you're vegetarian
- 1 little onion, finely chopped
- 3 garlic cloves, finely chopped
- ¼ tsp turmeric
- ½ tsp garam masala
- coriander, to serve
- 1 little tomato, chopped

Strategy:

1. Wash the lentils a few times until the water runs clear, at that point tip into a pan with 1 liter water and a touch of salt. Bring to the bubble, at that point diminish the heat and stew for 25 mins, skimming the foam from the

top. Cover with a top and cook for a further 40 mins, blending infrequently, until it's a thick, soupy consistency.
2. While the lentils are cooking, heat the ghee or oil in a non-stick skillet over a medium heat, at that point fry the onion and garlic until the onion is softened, so around 8 mins. Add the turmeric and garam masala, at that point cook briefly. Put away.
3. Tip the lentils into bowls and spoon a large portion of the onion blend on top. Top with the coriander and tomato to serve.
4. GOES WELL WITH
5. Spinach dhal with paneer
6. Bombay potato and spinach pies

26. potato dhal with curried vegetables

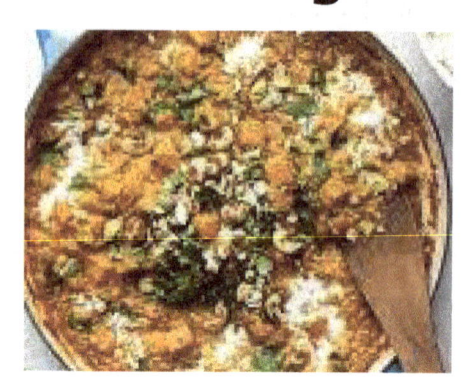

Prep:25 mins Cook:1 hr and 10 mins Easy
Serves 4

Ingredients:

- 1 tbsp cold-squeezed rapeseed oil
- 1 medium onion , finely chopped
- 2 garlic cloves , daintily cut
- 1 tbsp medium curry powder
- 200g dried split red lentils
- 500g yams , stripped and cut into pieces
- 2 tbsp lime (or lemon) juice in addition to lime wedges, to serve
- 100g full-fat characteristic bio yogurt
- coriander , to serve
- For the curried vegetables
- 100g green beans , managed and cut into off lengths

- 250g cauliflower, cut into little florets
- 2 medium carrots, cut
- 1 tbsp cold-squeezed rapeseed oil
- 1 medium onion, cut into slender wedges
- 2 garlic cloves, daintily cut
- 1 tsp medium curry powder
- 200g ready tomatoes, generally chopped
- 1 long green bean stew, finely cut (deseeded in the event that you don't care for it excessively hot)

Strategy:

1. To make the dhal, heat the oil in a large non-stick dish and fry the onion over a low heat for 10 mins, mixing consistently, until softened and gently browned – add the garlic for the last min. Mix in the curry powder and cook for 30 secs more.

2. Add the lentils, 1 tsp chipped ocean salt and 1 liter of water. Mix in the yams and bring to the bubble. Diminish the heat to a stew and cook the lentils for 50 mins or until the dhal is thick, blending consistently. Add a sprinkle of water if the dhal thickens excessively. Mix in the lime or lemon squeeze and season to taste.

3. While the dhal is cooking, make the curried vegetables. Half-fill a medium non-leave dish with water and bring to the bubble. Add the beans, cauliflower and carrots, and get back to the bubble. Cook for 4 mins, at that point channel.
4. Return the skillet to the heat and add the oil and onion. Cook over a medium-high heat for 3-4 mins or until the onion is gently browned, mixing routinely. Add the garlic and cook for 1 min more until softened. Mix in the curry powder and cook for a couple of secs, blending.
5. Add the tomatoes, green stew as indicated by taste and 200ml virus water. Cook for 5 mins or until the tomatoes are well softened, mixing routinely. Mix in the whitened vegetables and cook for 4-5 mins or until hot all through. Season with dark pepper.
6. Split the dhal between four profound dishes and top with the curried vegetables. Present with the yogurt, coriander and lime wedges for pressing over.
7. **Formula TIPS**
8. Putting away LEFTOVERS

9. Freeze the dhal and vegetables in lidded cooler confirmation holders for as long as 3 months. Defrost for the time being then add a sprinkle of water and reheat until steaming hot all through.

27. black dhal with crispy onions

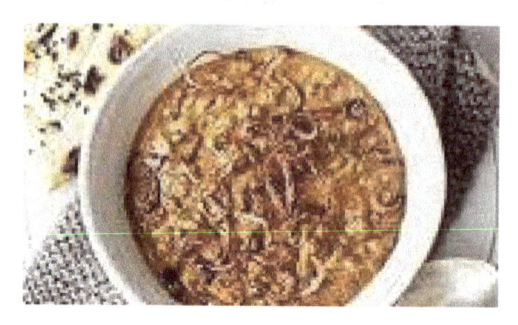

Prep:35 mins Cook:6 hrs and 35 mins plus 4 hrs soaking (cook for 2 hrs 35 mins, if using hob instead of slow cooker) Easy Serves 4

Ingredients:

- 250g dark urid beans (additionally called urid dal, urad dal, dark lentils or dark gram beans - accessible from large grocery stores) - yellow split peas likewise function admirably
- 100g margarine or ghee
- 2 large white onions, divided and meagerly cut
- 3 garlic cloves, squashed
- thumb-sized piece ginger, stripped and finely chopped
- 2 tsp ground cumin
- 2 tsp ground coriander
- 1 tsp ground turmeric
- 1 tsp paprika

- ¼ tsp bean stew powder (optional)
- little bundle coriander, follows finely chopped, leaves held to serve
- 400g passata or chopped tomatoes
- 1 fat red bean stew, punctured a couple of times with the tip of a sharp blade
- 50ml twofold cream
- To serve
- cooked rice, naan bread or heated yams
- coriander
- cut red bean stew
- lime wedges
- yogurt (or a twirl of cream)
- your #1 Indian pickle or chutney
- firm plate of mixed greens onions (to make your own, see formula beneath)

Technique:
1. Absorb the beans cold water for 4 hrs (or overnight, on the off chance that you like).
2. Soften the margarine or ghee in a large dish, at that point add the onions, garlic and ginger, and cook gradually for 10-15 mins until the onions are beginning to caramelize. Mix in the flavors, coriander stalks and 100ml water. Fill

the sluggish cooker (or leave in the skillet if cooking on the hob). Add the passata and entire red stew. Channel the beans and add these as well, at that point top up with 400ml water. Season well, set the sluggish cooker to Low and cook for 5-6 hrs (or cover and cook for 2 hrs over an exceptionally low heat on the hob).

3. When cooked, the dhal ought to be exceptionally thick and the beans delicate. Mix in the cream, check the flavoring and serve in bowls with naan bread, rice or in a coat potato, with your selection of garnishes. To freeze the dhal, cool totally, at that point partition into compartments or sandwich sacks. Freeze for as long as 2 months, thaw out and heat altogether prior to eating.
4. **Formula TIPS**
5. TO MAKE THE CRISPY ONIONS
6. Meagerly cut 1 red or white onion. Heat sufficient vegetable or sunflower oil to come 1-2 cm up the side of a large skillet. When hot, fry the onions in groups until fresh, channel on kitchen paper and sprinkle with salt.

28. Mild split pea & spinach dhal

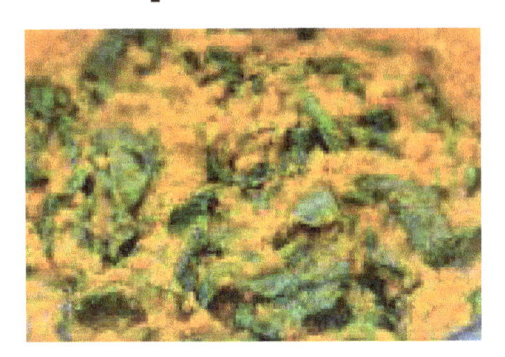

Prep:10 mins Cook:1 hr and 15 mins Easy Makes 5 toddler portions

Ingredients:

- 175g yellow split peas
- ½ tbsp coconut oil
- 1 little onion , finely chopped
- 1 fat garlic clove , squashed
- ½ tsp yellow mustard seeds
- ¼ tsp turmeric
- 1 ½ tsp gentle curry powder
- 50g unsalted cashew nuts , chopped
- 1 low salt vegetable stock 3D square (we utilized Kallo)
- 100g frozen chopped spinach
- plain yogurt , pitta bread or rice, to serve

Technique:

1. Absorb the yellow split peas a bowl of water for 20 mins. Flush completely in a couple of changes of water.
2. Heat the oil in a large hefty based pan. Cook the onion for 5-10 mins, mixing every now and then until softened and beginning to caramelize. Add the garlic and flavors and cook for a further 1-2 mins permitting the fragrances to deliver.
3. Heartbeat the cashews in a food processor into fine pieces – ensure you do this well so that there is no danger of gagging. Add the split peas and cashews to the skillet, at that point pour in sufficient water to cover it by a couple of cms. Disintegrate in the veg stock 3D square. Bring to the bubble, at that point stew for 1hr or until the split peas are delicate, mixing every now and then. In the event that they begin to look somewhat dry, include more water depending on the situation during the cooking. Mix through the frozen chopped spinach and once the dhal is hot all through, present with a spot of yogurt on top, pitta or brown rice.
4. GOES WELL WITH

5. Little child formula: Mini shepherd's pies
6. Little child formula: Chicken cashew satay on lolly sticks
7. Little child formula: Mini egg and veg biscuits

29. Makhani dhal

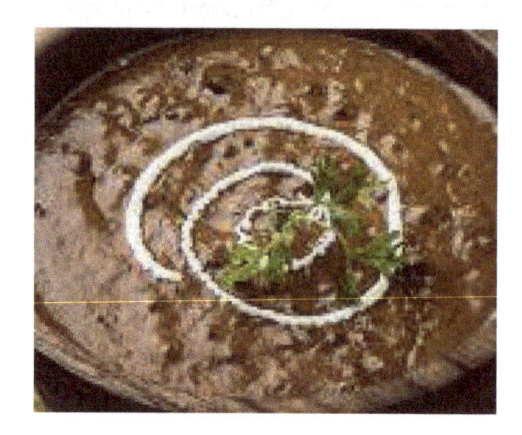

Prep:10 mins Cook:45 mins Easy Serves 8

Ingredients:

- 225g dark lentils
- 2 onions , finely chopped
- 2 green chillies , deseeded and cut
- 50g margarine , in addition to a little lump
- 1 tbsp ground new root ginger
- 3 garlic cloves , meagerly cut
- 1 tsp ground turmeric
- ½ tsp hot bean stew powder (optional)
- 2 tsp ground cumin
- 2 tsp ground coriander
- 2 narrows leaves
- 2 x 400g jars red kidney beans , flushed
- 142ml pot twofold cream
- ½ tsp garam masala

- modest bunch chopped coriander

Technique:

1. Heat up the lentils in 800ml water for 15 mins until practically delicate. Then, fry the onions and chillies in the 50g margarine for around 7 mins until beginning to mellow. Mix in the ginger, garlic and flavors and cook over a low heat for 1 min more.
2. Pour in 800ml bubbling water followed by the cooked lentils and any fluid. Add the straight leaves and beans, at that point stew for 20 mins more until thickened. This can be made 2 days ahead and chilled, or frozen for as long as multi month.
3. To serve, get back to the heat if important and mix in the cream. Season well. Fill a bowl, spot with the excess margarine, dust with garam masala and disperse with coriander.

30. Tomatoes stuffed with fruity dhal

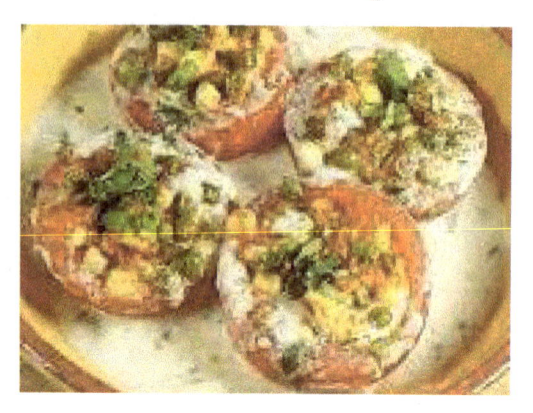

Prep:15 mins Cook:50 mins Easy

Ingredients:

- 100ml yellow split pea
- 2 ½ tbsp sunflower oil
- 1 little onion , finely chopped
- 2 garlic cloves , squashed
- 1 tsp cayenne pepper
- 1 tsp turmeric
- 50g raisin
- 100g cooked chickpea
- 2 tbsp mango chutney
- 2 tbsp chopped new coriander
- 4 large meat tomatoes

Strategy:

1. Put the split peas in a container with 600ml/1pt virus water. Bring to the bubble and skim the surface to eliminate any filth. Diminish the heat and stew for 20 mins. Heat oven to 190C/fan 170C/gas 5.
2. In the mean time, heat 2 tbsp of the oil in a skillet and cook the onion and garlic for 4 mins until softened. Mix in the flavors, at that point cook briefly. Mix this blend and the raisins into the split peas, at that point cook for a further 10 mins until delicate and velvety. Mix in the chickpeas, chutney and coriander and heat through. Season to taste.
3. Cut the tops off the hamburger tomatoes and save. Scratch out the internal parts and dispose of. Spoon the dhal blend into the tomatoes and supplant the tops. Spot on a heating sheet and brush with the leftover oil. Cook for 20 mins until the tomatoes have softened.

31. halloumi fritters with coriander dip

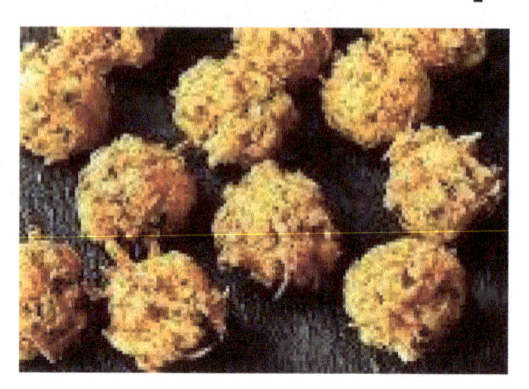

Prep:30 mins Cook:20 mins Serves 12

Ingredients:

- 1 egg, beaten
- 60g plain flour
- 1 onion, coarsely ground
- 4 carrots, coarsely ground
- 250g halloumi, coarsely ground
- thumb-sized piece of ginger, stripped and finely ground
- 1 red bean stew, finely chopped
- 2 tsp ground coriander
- little bundle of coriander, finely chopped
- vegetable oil, for browning
- For the coriander plunge
- 200g Greek yogurt
- 4 tbsp margarine or ghee

- ½ tsp smoked paprika
- spot of stew chips
- ½ tbsp coriander seeds, squashed

Technique:

1. Whisk the egg and flour together in a large bowl until thick and irregularity free, at that point crease in the onion, carrots, halloumi, ginger, stew, ground coriander, a large portion of the new coriander and a lot of preparing. The combination ought to be very solid – if the hitter isn't covering the veg, add another tablespoon of flour or a little sprinkle of milk.

2. Fill a medium weighty based pan close to a third loaded with vegetable oil and heat to 180C, or until a solid shape of bread sizzles when dropped into the oil, and browns in around 30 seconds.

3. Structure the waste combination into scaled down balls using your hands or two little spoons. Fry the squanders in clusters of five or six, turning in the oil at regular intervals for an aggregate of 5-6 mins, or until fresh and golden brown. Channel on kitchen paper and serve hot, or leave to cool and reheat prior to

serving. Will keep in a water/air proof compartment in the ice chest for as long as three days, or in the cooler for a quarter of a year. To reheat, heat the oven to 220C/200C fan/gas 7, move to a preparing plate, and prepare for 5-10 mins until fresh and heated through.

4. To make the plunge, consolidate the yogurt, the greater part of the leftover new coriander, and some flavoring. Dissolve the margarine or ghee in a little skillet, at that point mix in the paprika, bean stew drops and coriander seeds. Sizzle for 1 min, at that point pour over the yogurt. Top with the remainder of the coriander, and present with the wastes for dunking.

Conclusion

I would like to thank you for choosing this book .Hope you liked all recipes. These have main ingredients coconut which provides alkalinity in body and it also has certain health benefits. Prepare and enjoy
I wish you good luck!

CPSIA information can be obtained
at www.ICGtesting.com
Printed in the USA
BVHW092125090621
609092BV00002B/587